NAVIGATING THE MIND:
A journey through mental health

By

AUGUSTINE OLISEL|KALU
SPECIAL

TABLE OF CONTENTS

INTRODUCTION: 4

CHAPTER ONE: Understanding Mental Health............... 5

- Defining Mental Health................................. 5
- Common Misconceptions............................. 7
- Importance of Mental Well-being.................... 8

CHAPTER TWO: Breaking the Stigma....................... 10

- Addressing Societal Stigmas......................... 11
- Overcoming Self-Stigma............................... 13
- Advocating for Change................................. 15

CHAPTER THREE: Types of Mental Health Disorders...... 18

CHAPTER FOUR: Personal Stories of Resilience.......... 21

- Interview individuals sharing their Journeys......... 22
- Overcoming Challenges................................ 24

CHAPTER FIVE: Seeking Help................................. 27

CHAPTER SIX: Building Mental Resilience.................. 29

CHAPTER SEVEN: Relationships and Mental Health...... 31

- Impact of Relationships on Mental Well-being...... 31
- Communicating about Mental Health................. 32
- Supportive Networks................................... 33

CHAPTER EIGHT: Navigating Mental Health at Work...... 37

- Creating a Healthy Work Environment................ 37
- Balancing Work and Well-being....................... 39

CHAPTER NINE: Future Perspectives........................41
- Advancements in Mental Health Research.........42
- Shaping a More Inclusive Society..................43

CONCLUSION: 45
- Encouragement and Hope...........................46
- Call to Action..48

INTRODUCTION

Welcome to "Navigating the Mind: A Journey Through Mental Health." In these pages, we embark on a fascinating journey through the depth of consciousness and emotions. From the depth of communication and enriching understanding of everyday emotions to the hidden opportunities for growth and discovery on mental health conditions, this book offers a compassionate exploration of the dynamic realm where our hopes, dreams, and memory reside. Join me as we delve into the complexities of the mind, understanding the multitude of perspectives, backgrounds and identities that shape an individual's life, struggles, and achievement that define our mental health journeys. Together, let us embark on a journey through countless pathways full of unexpected detours and surprises, building strong communities and individuals.

CHAPTER ONE
UNDERSTANDING MENTAL HEALTH

Mental health is a crucial aspect of feeling content and satisfied with life, influencing how we perceive and interact with the world, psychological, and social factors. It is influenced by a combination of genetic, environmental, and lifestyle factors. Understanding mental health involves recognizing the importance of addressing issues such as stress, anxiety, depression, and other disorders. Promoting mental health awareness, reducing stigma, and seeking support when needed are essential for maintaining optimal mental well-being. By organizing tasks and goals based on the importance of mental health, individuals can lead fulfilling lives and contribute positively to their communities.

DEFINING MENTAL HEALTH

Mental health refers to a person's emotional, psychological, and social well-being. It includes how individuals think, feel, and behave, and it impacts how they handle stress, relate to others, and make choices. Mental health is not just the absence of mental illness but also the presence of positive qualities, resilience, and the ability to cope with life's challenges effectively. It can also be defined as a state of wellbeing in which an individual realizes their own potential, cope with the normal stresses of life, work productively, and contribute to their community. In other words mental health is fundamental to total fitness, embracing emotional, psychological, and social aspects. It exceeds the absence of mental illness, displaying determination, positive qualities, and successful adaptation strategy. A key aspect of mental health is the realization of one's potential and the ability to guide life challenges while maintaining productivity and contributing positively to society. Access to resources and support systems holds significant importance promoting and maintaining mental well-being, specifically connected to physical health.

COMMON MISCONCEPTIONS

Common Misconceptions About Mental Health;

1. Children don't experience mental health issues: children can experience mental health issues just like adults. These issues might manifest differently due to their developmental stage, but conditions like anxiety, depression, ADHD, and behavioral disorders can affect children too. It's important to recognize and address these issues early to provide proper support and treatment.

2. Therapy is only for people with severe mental illnesses: Therapy is beneficial for various mental health concerns, from everyday stress to diagnosable disorders, and can help individuals develop plan to achieve and improve their overall well-being.

3. People with mental illnesses are violent or dangerous: Most people with mental illness are not violent. Mental health conditions vary greatly in their symptoms and complex, and the majority of individuals living with them are peaceful and law-abiding.

4. You can always tell when someone is struggling with their mental health: Mental health challenges are not always visible, and individuals may be an expert at hiding their struggles. It's important to be supportive and nonjudgmental.

5. Once you're cured, you'll never have to worry about mental health again: Mental health is a constant aspect of overall well-being, and individuals may experience periods of stability as well as times of difficulty throughout their lives. Ongoing self-care and support are essential for maintaining good mental health.

IMPORTANCE OF MENTAL WELL-BEING

In today's fast-paced world, mental well-being is not just an enjoyable pleasure but a basic requirement for human well being. Just as we determine the importance of our physical health, we must also care for our minds. Mental well-being encompasses emotional, psychological, and social health, impacting every aspect of our lives. It affects how we think, feel, and act, influencing our relationships, work performance, and overall quality of life. Maintaining good mental well-being involves self-care practices such as regular exercise, adequate sleep, healthy eating, and stress management techniques. It also involves seeking support when needed, either from friends, family, or mental health professionals. By acknowledging and addressing our mental health needs, we can lead more fulfilling lives and contribute positively to our communities. Remember, focusing on our mental well-being is not a sign of weakness but of strength. It's okay not to be okay sometimes, and seeking help is a courageous step toward healing and growth. Let's work together to break the shame surrounding mental health and create a culture where everyone feels supported and valued.

CHAPTER TWO
BREAKING THE STIGMA

In recent years, there has been a growing recognition of the importance of mental health and the need to break the negative attitude surrounding it. This belief often prevents individuals from seeking help and support when they need it most. By cultivating open conversations, promoting understanding, and providing accessible resources, we can create a society where mental health is treated as important as physical health.

Breaking the stigma around mental health likely involves exacting negative attitudes, beliefs, and stereotypes that lead to discrimination and restrain people from seeking help. It requires nurturing understanding and empathy, acceptance of mental health conditions as valid health considerations just like physical illnesses. This can be achieved through education, open conversations, sharing personal experiences, and promoting access to mental health services without fear of judgement or discrimination.

Ultimately, overcoming misconceptions requires collective efforts to create a supportive and universal environment where everyone feels comfortable addressing their mental health needs.

ADDRESSING SOCIETAL STIGMA

Addressing societal stigma on mental health requires different aspects of approach involving education, support, and empathy. Here is a structured approach to address this stigma:

1. **Education and Awareness**: Promoting the understanding of mental health conditions through education campaigns, workshops, and media outreach. Recognizing the frequency and wide range of mental illnesses to expose myths and stereotypes.

2. **Encourage Open Dialogue:** Create safe spaces for discussing mental health openly without being judgmental. Encourage individuals to share their experiences, fostering empathy, understanding and cooperation.

3. **Combat Language Stigma:** Encourage the use of respectful and non stigmatizing language when discussing mental health. Avoid critical

terms that diminish or belittle the worth of a person or group and give accurate attention on respecting the individual's humility and not focus on their disability.

4. Empowerment through Representation: Increase representation of diverse mental health experiences in media, literature, and popular culture. Emphasizing on stories of recovery and adapting solemnly on trauma to inspire hope and reduce feelings of loneliness.

5. **Accessible Support Services:** Ensure access to affordable and culturally capable mental health services for all individuals. This includes increasing funding for mental health programs and improving access to care in underserved communities.

6. **Train Healthcare Providers:** Provide training for healthcare professionals to recognize and address mental health stigma in clinical settings. Encourage a comprehensive approach to healthcare that ranks mental well-being alongside physical health.

7. **Legislation and Policy Reform:** Advocate for policies that protect the rights of individuals with mental illnesses and promote integration in all aspects of society. This includes

antidiscrimination laws and workplace accommodations for individuals with mental health conditions.

8. **Community Support and Involvement:** Engage communities to act independently to reduce mental health stigma. Encourage teamwork between local organizations, schools, businesses, and religiously oriented groups to create supportive environments for those affected by mental illness.

By implementing these strategies, we can work towards creating a more compassionate and welcoming society where mental health is prioritized and stigma is minimized.

OVERCOMING SELF-STIGMA

Overcoming self-stigma on mental health involves several steps:

1. **Educate Yourself:** Learn and have ideas about mental health conditions, their causes, and treatments.

Understanding that mental illnesses are medical conditions can help reduce self-stigma.

2. **Challenge Negative Beliefs:** Recognize and challenge negative beliefs about yourself and your mental health. Replace them with positive affirmations and compassionate selftalk. Make yourself busy, creating no time for negative thoughts.

3. **Seek Support:** Talk to friends, family, or a therapist about your feelings and experiences. Connecting with others who understand and accept you the way you are can reduce feelings of loneliness and selfdiscrimination.

4. **Practice Self-Compassion:** Treat yourself with kindness, put yourself as a priority. Acknowledge that struggling with mental health does not make you weak or inferior to others.

5. **Set Realistic Goals:** Break tasks into manageable steps and celebrate your achievements, bring your thoughts into reality, no matter how small. Building confidence and self-esteem can neutralize feelings of self-stigma.

6. **Focus on Strengths:** Identify and focus on your strengths and accomplishments. Recognize that mental illness does not define you as a

person, neither does it stop you from getting to a higher length of learning.

7. **Advocate for Yourself:** Speak up against discrimination and stigma in your community. By supporting yourself and others, you can help break down stereotypes and promote acceptance.

8. **Practice Self-Care:** Prioritize activities that promote your mental and emotional well-being, such as exercise, meditation, hobbies, and spending time with loved ones.

Remember, overcoming self-stigma is a journey, and it's okay to seek professional help if needed. You are not alone, and there is hope for recovery and acceptance.

ADVOCATING FOR CHANGE

1. **Educate Yourself:** Before advocating for change, educate yourself on the current state of mental health, including statistics, common issues, and existing resources. Understanding the key elements and dynamics will help you advocate more effectively.

2. **Raise Awareness:** Use your voice and platform to raise consciousness about mental

health issues. Share personal stories, statistics, and information about available resources to help educate others and reduce stigma.

3. **Engage with Decision-Makers:** Reach out to policymakers, government officials, and community leaders to advocate for policies and enterprises that support mental health. Send messages, make phone calls, and attend town hall meetings to express your concerns and urge for change.

4. **Promote Mental Wellness Initiatives:** Support and promote initiatives that focus on mental wellness and prevention, such as mental health education programs in schools, workplace wellness motivation, and community support groups.

5. **Advocate for Accessible Mental Health Care:** Advocate for increased access to affordable mental health care services, including therapy, counselling, and psychiatric care. Support policies that expand mental health scope and funding for mental health programs.

6. **Challenge Stigma:** Challenge stigma and discrimination surrounding mental illness by promoting open conversations and understanding. Encourage people to seek help

without fear of judgement and speak out against harmful stereotypes and misconceptions.

7. **Collaborate with Others:** Join forces with like-minded individuals and organizations that are also advocating for change in mental health. Cooperating with others can enhance your efforts and make a greater impact.

8. **Use Social Media:** Apply social media platforms to spread awareness, share resources, and assemble support for mental health advocacy. Use hashtags, create online campaigns, and engage with others to spark conversations and advance change.

By following these steps and staying persistent in your advocacy efforts, you can help drive positive change and improve the state of mental health in your community and beyond.

CHAPTER THREE

TYPE OF MENTAL HEALTH DISORDERS

A mental disorder, also known as a mental illness, is a condition defining qualities by significant disturbances in a person's thoughts, emotions, or behaviors, leading to extreme sorrow, pain or reduced capacity in daily life. Mental health disorders include a wide variety of conditions that affect mood, thinking, and behavior. Some major types include:

1. **Anxiety disorders:** these are a group of mental health conditions defined by excessive worry, fear, or nervousness. They can manifest as generalized anxiety disorder, panic disorder, social anxiety disorder, specific phobias, and others. Symptoms include restlessness, irritation, muscle tension, difficulty concentrating, and sleep disturbances. Treatment includes therapy, medication, and lifestyle changes to help manage symptoms and improve quality of life.

2. **Mood disorders:** There are mental health conditions that mainly affect a person's emotional state. Conditions such as depression, bipolar disorder, and cyclothymic disorder.

Symptoms can change widely but often involve preserving feelings of sadness, hopelessness, irritability, or mood swings. Treatment involves a combination of therapy, medication, and lifestyle changes to balance mood and improve general well-being.

3. **Psychotic disorders:** Involve significant disturbances in awareness, thoughts, emotions, and behavior. They can cause individuals to detach from reality, experiencing delusions, uncoordinated thinking, and diminished social functioning. Treatment often involves a combination of medication, therapy, and support services.

4. **Eating disorder:** it is a mental health condition characterized by irregular eating habits and excessive discomfort or concern about body weight or shape. There are several types of eating disorders, including anorexia nervosa (restricting food intake to lose weight), bulimia nervosa (binge eating followed by purging behaviors), and binge eating disorder (frequent episodes of consuming large amounts of food without control). These disorders can have serious physical and emotional consequences and often require professional treatment.

5. **Substance use disorder (SUD):** It's a medical condition identified by a determined pattern of challenging use of a substance, leading to significant limitations or afflictions. It's often associated with tolerance (needing more of the substance to achieve the same effect) and abstinence effect when not using the substance. SUD can affect various aspects of a person's life, including their physical health, mental well-being, relationships, and ability to play a role in daily life.

CHAPTER FOUR
PERSONAL STORY OF RESILIENCE

Growing up, I faced many challenges, but one of the most challenging occurred during the period of financial struggle my family faced. My parents were unemployed due to job loss, we struggled to make ends meet. Despite the confusions and stress, my parents never gave up. They worked part time, applied for assistance programs, and did every possible thing they could to provide for the family.

Having seen their persistence in moving forward, it inspired me to persevere through my own challenges. I worked hard in school, applied for scholarships, and took on part-time jobs to help relieve the financial burden on my family. It wasn't easy at the beginning, but through determination I refused to let circumstances define my future.

Eventually, the situation improved. My parents found stable employment, and

I graduated from college with honors.

Looking back, I realize our perseverance during those tough times formed who I am today. It taught me the importance of perseverance, determination, and never losing hope, even in the face of challenges.

INTERVIEWS WITH INDIVIDUALS SHARING THEIR JOURNEY

Here are some experts from interviews with individuals sharing their journey:

1. **Entrepreneurial Journey:** Starting my own business was a bold move. I faced countless challenges along the way, but each challenge taught me irreplaceable lessons about endurance and determination. Building something from the ground up is incredibly rewarding, despite the obstacles.

2. **Career Transition:** Transforming to a new career path was intimidating, but I knew I needed to pursue my passion. It required perseverance and a willingness to learn, but eventually, it was worth it. Embracing change revealed new opportunities I never imagined."

3. **Personal Growth:** Embarking on a journey of self-discovery was transformative. It meant confronting my fears and insecurities, but through self-reflection, I reached a greater level of insight of myself. Embracing my weakness allowed me to cultivate meaningful connections and lead a more genuine life.

4. **Overcoming Adversity:** Facing challenges tested my endurance in ways I never imagined. Whether it was overcoming illness, loss, or failure, each setback I faced grew my determination. Through perseverance and a positive mindset, I learned to turn obstacles into opportunities for growth.

5. **Creative Pursuits:** Pursuing my creative passions has been both challenging and fulfilling. It's required dedication, discipline, and a willingness to take risks. But seeing my ideas and opinions come to reality and connecting with others through expression has been incredibly rewarding." Each individual's journey is unique, shaped by their experiences, choices, and perseverance.

OVERCOMING CHALLENGES

Here are some practical strategies to overcome challenges related to mental health:

1. **Seek Professional Help:** Seek advice from a mental health professional, such as a therapist or counsellor, who can provide guidance, support, and counselling methods personalized to your specific needs.

2. **Build a Support Network:** Surround yourself with supportive friends, family members, or helpful groups who can offer empathy, understanding, and encouragement during difficult times.

3. **Practice Self-Care:** Organize selfcare activities that promote physical, emotional, and mental well-being, such as regular exercise, healthy eating, adequate sleep, and relaxation techniques like meditation or deep breathing exercises.

4. **Develop Coping Skills:** Learn and practice healthy adaptation to manage stress, anxiety, and other symptoms associated with mental health . These challenges include mindfulness, record keeping, creative expression, or engaging in activities that bring you happiness.

5. **Set Realistic Goals:** Disintegrate large goals into smaller, achievable steps, and celebrate your achievement and progress along the way. Setting realistic expectations for yourself helps prevent feelings of defeat and boosts self-confidence.

6. **Establish Routine:** Create a daily routine that includes organization and consistency, as this can provide a sense of stability and reliability, which are critical for symptom regulation of mental health conditions.

7. **Challenge Negative Thoughts:** Practice mental-behavioral techniques to identify and challenge negative thought patterns or beliefs that support the feelings of distress or self-doubt. Substitute them with more positive and realistic interpretation.

8. **Stay Connected:** Maintain social connections, involving in activities that cultivate a consciousness of belonging and connecting with others. Loneliness and exclusion can worsen mental health challenges, making an effort to stay connected with loved ones.

9. **Limit Stressors:** Identify sources of stress in your daily life and take preventive steps to reduce or eliminate them when possible. This

involves setting boundaries, assigning tasks, or seeking professional support to address foundational issues.

10. **Practice Patience and SelfCompassion:** Being patient with yourself directs the ups and downs of your mental health journey. Treat yourself with kindness, compassion, and understanding, accepting that healing takes time and effort.

Remember, everyone's journey to overcome mental health challenges is extraordinarily different, so it's crucial to find strategies and approaches that work best for you. Don't hesitate to reach out for help and support when needed, and remember that recovery is possible with perseverance.

CHAPTER FIVE
SEEKING HELP

Seeking help for mental health is an important step towards well-being. Here's a guide:

1. **Recognizing signs of mental health issues:** these involve observing changes in behavior, mood, or thinking patterns. These include increased irritability, withdrawal from social activities, changes in sleep or appetite, excessive worry, mood swings, and difficulty concentrating. If you notice these signs continuously or affecting daily functioning, it may indicate a need for professional help.

2. **Professional support:** it's fundamental for mental health due to its provision of expertise, guidance, and customized treatment options that individuals may not have access to alternatively. Professionals can offer a safe space for expressing emotions, adaptive techniques, and prescribe medications if needed, all of which can considerably improve mental wellbeing.

3. Therapy in the background of mental health, which involves meeting with a professional to address emotional, psychological, or behavioral

issues. It can take various forms such as talk therapy, mental-behavioral therapy, or medication management. The purpose 1 is to provide support, guidance, and strategies to help individuals confront and overcome their challenges.

Therapy sessions typically involve open dialogue, exploration of thoughts and feelings, and the development of dealing with the system adapting to the individual's needs.

Remember, seeking help is a courageous and important step towards healing and well-being. You're not alone, and there are people and resources available to support you.

CHAPTER SIX
BUILDING MENTAL RESILIENCE

Building mental strength is essential for guiding life's challenges with grace and strength. Here are some schemes to improve steadfastness:

1.**Self-care for mental health requires organized practices that nurture emotional well-being and inner strength:** This includes determining physical health, setting boundaries, developing emotional intelligence, participating in pleasurable activities, practicing mindfulness and relaxation methods, reaching out for assistance, and being approachable to professional help when needed. By applying these strategies into your daily schedule, you can promote mental well-being and upgrade the ability to deal with life's challenges. Remember, self-care is essential for maintaining balance and energy in all aspects of life.

2. **Meditation involves training your mind to focus and guide your thoughts:** It can help reduce stress and anxiety, develop concentration, and advance emotional well-being. Reflection is a type of meditation that involves the

concentration on the current moment without being judged. Both routines have been shown to benefit mental health by decreasing symptoms of depression, anxiety, and other mental health conditions.

3. **Maintaining a healthy lifestyle is fundamental for mental well-being:** These include regular exercise, balanced nutrition, adequate rest, stress reduction methods such as listening to music, nurturing supportive relationships, and engaging in enjoyable activities. These procedures help to reduce stress, boost emotional well being, improve mental abilities , and build inner strength.

CHAPTER SEVEN
RELATIONSHIP AND MENTAL HEALTH

Relationships and mental care are interconnected at a fundamental level. In a relationship, it's important to be focused on mental well-being for both companions. These involve open communication, compassion, and understanding each other's emotions and needs. Mental care within a relationship includes supporting each other during difficult times, developing attentive listening, and seeking professional help if needed. Taking care of one's mental health also supplies to the health of the relationship, it allows individuals to be more impartial, patient, and compassionate towards each other.

IMPACT OF RELATIONSHIP ON MENTAL WELL-BEING

Relationships have a meaningful impact on mental well-being. Beneficial relationships can provide emotional support, decrease feelings of loneliness, and increase happiness and satisfaction. They provide a feeling of connection and security, which can safeguard against stress and anxiety. Alternatively, unfavorable or unhealthy relationships can heighten the sensation of discomfort, stimulate low self-esteem, and depression. Harmful relationship patterns, such as lack of communication, manipulation, or emotional abuse, worsen mental health issues. Hence, nurturing healthy relationships built on trust, respect, and mutual support is essential for maintaining and improving mental well-being.

COMMUNICATING ABOUT MENTAL

Communicating about mental health involves uttering your feelings and experiences transparently and honestly, while also attentive and compassionate listening to others. It's significant to use open minded languages, acknowledging and affirm others feelings, and present support without trying to resolve their problems. Additionally, increasing consciousness, educating yourself and others, and supporting mental health resources and services can help eliminate social disgrace and promote understanding.

Furthermore, mental health is essential for increasing understanding, encouraging empathy and promoting support for individuals experiencing mental health challenges. It involves discussing topics such as depression, anxiety, bipolar disorder, PTSD, and more, in a compassionate and open approach. Effective communication on mental health includes listening actively, respecting reaction, extending assistance, and encouraging individuals to seek professional help when needed.

It's also important to use respectful language, avoid stereotypes, and protect sensitive information to create a safe and supportive environment for discussion.

SUPPORTIVE NETWORK

Building supportive networks for mental health involves surrounding yourself with understanding and passionate individuals who are eager to attend without judgement. These networks can include friends, family members, support groups, therapists, or online communities.

In navigating the advanced environment of mental health, benefiting from a comprehensive and supportive system that includes a wide range of resources, individuals, and communities that universally extend empathy, encouragement, and

practical assistance

to those dealing with mental health challenges.

Basically, a support network is about stimulating connections with others who understand your experiences are devoted to your well-being. This network can include family members and close friends who provide constant emotional support, offering a supportive presence and providing comfort during difficult times. Their open minded presence can serve as a source of comfort and affirmation of feeling, helping to diminish feelings of withdrawal and loneliness.

Mental health professionals, such as therapists, counsellors, and psychiatrists, are essential components of a support network. These trained professionals provide specialised knowledge in guiding mental health issues, developing specialized therapy programs, survival methods, and research supported approaches . Their guidance strengthens individuals to challenge their difficulties with endurance and determination, encouraging a sense of hope and growth along their journey of healing.

Support groups and performance based platforms create an irreplaceable environment for individuals to engage in social interaction sharing similar experiences. These groups provide a feeling of inclusion and understanding, creating a supportive environment where individuals can share their stories, exchange advice, and find empowerment through collective wisdom. Regardless of the setting, support groups encourage a bond of companionship and unity, affirming the idea that everyone is supported in their struggles.

In the age of technology online resources and call centres create easy reachable part forms seeking support and information. Online platforms, discussion boards and support lines offer an abundance of information, including educational materials, personal development resources and opportunities for private peer assistance. These platforms overcome distance limitations and provide uninterrupted assistance at all hours, ensuring that help is available whenever it's needed.

Building a support network is an active and continuous progression that requires honesty, trust, and sensitivity. It's about making connections with others, developing genuine relationships, and acknowledging the power of unity in the community. Dedicating resources to complex connections, individuals can develop inner strength, promote recovery, commence on an adventure towards mental well-being with confidence and courage.

In essence, a support network for mental health is a guiding light in dark times, compassion, and understanding in the regularly demanding territory of mental illness. It serves as a reminder that no one should progress through their journey alone together we can overcome hardship and effort.

CHAPTER EIGHT

NAVIGATING MENTAL HEALTH AT WORK

Guiding Mental health at work involves ordering self-care, establishing limits, reaching out for assistance from colleagues or professionals, and communicating honestly with your director about your needs. It's decisive to detect weariness indicators of stress and take initiative steps to address them, such as taking breaks, engaging in the present moment and seeking residence as circumstances dictate.

CREATING A HEALTHY WORK ENVIRONMENT

Creating a healthy work environment for mental health involves several methods:

1. **Promote Open Communication:** Inspire employees to speak honestly about mental health challenges with complete freedom from judgement or consequences.

2. **Provide Resources:** Provide approach to mental health resources such as counselling services, support groups, or workshops.

3. **Training and Education:** Provide instructions to managers and employees on recognizing signs of mental health issues and how to support colleagues in need of assistance.

4. **Flexible Policies:** Introduce work schedules, such as home based employment or customizable hours to accommodate individuals dealing with mental health challenges.

5. **Normalize Self-Care:** Promote breaks, vacations, and time off to re energize, by doing this techniques it encourages the culture of work life harmony.

6. **Lead by Example:** Managers and leaders should highlight their own mental health and illustrate healthy work-life balance.

7. **Promote Work-Life Balance:** Encourage employees to focus on their well-being at their leisure time, such as spending time with family, exploring personal interest and engaging in selfcare activities.

8. **Address Workplace Stressors:** Recognize and resolve workplace pressures, such as overwhelming amounts of tasks, poor communication, or lack of resources, that may contribute to poor mental health.

By incorporating these strategies into action, organizations can create a supportive and a welcoming atmosphere that embraces diversity and promotes inclusive emphasis on mental health and well-being.

BALANCING WORK AND WELLBEING

Balancing work and well-being is the maintenance of good mental health. It's vital to define clear limits, placing self care as a top concern, and articulate your needs clearly with your employer. Pausing for a moment of rest, exercising, and cultivating present moment awareness which can also help manage stress and maintain a healthy work-life balance.

Furthermore, it's essential for maintaining good mental health.

Organizing self-care activities such as exercise, stress relief methods, and spending time with loved ones can help manage tension. Setting boundaries around workplace engagement, and learning to say no when necessary, can prevent being exhausted. Self reflection and seeking support from colleagues or mental health professionals when needed are important steps in maintaining a healthy work-life balance. Ultimately, identifying your well-being is just as important as your work responsibilities is an essential element for maintaining unity.

CHAPTER NINE
FUTURE PERSPECTIVE

In the future, mental health is likely to become better incorporated into global health coverage, with intense concentration on prevention, early intervention, and personalised treatment approaches. Technology could play an important contribution, with advancements in artificial intelligence (AI), virtual environment, and personal accessories enhancing treatment plan, and monitoring. There may also be a transition towards a trouble-free environment, leading to transparent communication and greater societal support for those seeking help.

Additionally, it implies a movement in the direction of forward thinking methods and personalized approaches, exploiting developments in technology for early identification, unique interventions, and acceptance through increased recognition and understanding.

Additionally, incorporating mental health care into various aspects of life, such as education, work, and community support systems, is making progress for promoting overall wellbeing.

ADVANCEMENTS IN MENTAL HEALTH RESEARCH

Progress in mental health research is ongoing, with remarkable progress in areas such as understanding the brain's system, developing more effective therapies, and promoting understanding and acceptance surrounding mental health issues. Methods like mental replication and genetic research have further our insight of conditions like depression, schizophrenia, and PTSD clearing the path for more targeted treatments and involvement. Additionally, digital mental health digital counselling resources are increasing accessibility to care and support for individuals worldwide. Expanding one's understanding of advancement and growth in mental health research, We expect an enduring commitment to attention and focus progressing towards treatment designed for each individual needs and family trait. This involves additional incorporation of genetic information and artificial intelligence training to project the progress in treatment and specific guidance.

Additionally, development in brain imaging technology indicates potential for improved understanding of the basic process supporting various mental health disorders, leading to the development of more purposeful interventions.

Furthermore, the increased appreciation of the importance of complete care measures to mental health, including lifestyle factors such as diet, exercise, and social support, positioned to guide future research directions. The combined efforts between researchers, clinicians, and policymakers is essential for translating scientific discoveries to improved mental health results for individuals worldwide.

SHAPING A MORE INCLUSIVE SOCIETY

Creating affordable options for mental health resources for all individuals, normalizing conversation about mental health struggles around mental illness, and incorporating mental health education into various aspects of society such as schools, workplaces, and community programs. Additionally, creating opportunities for shared experience and connections, understanding, and support for those with mental health challenges can help create a culture of acceptance and participation. Creating space for voice from all backgrounds and experiences within mental health discussions can lead to more effective interventions and support systems for everyone.

CONCLUSION

In conclusion, exploring into the detail of the mind, the conclusion highlights the importance of encouraging an understanding of emotional health and mental well-being.

The narrative intentionally shifts his focus towards promoting the elimination of societal judgement of mental health, exploring into the complexities of your mind. It displays an inspiring image of courage and unwavering strength overcoming obstacles, in the face of adversity , the journey echoes the inner strength.

With each unfolding chapter a resounding theme emerges: the transformative force of self compassion.

As the book comes to an end it stands as an impassioned call to action by readers to extend kindness to themselves as they guide through the twists and turns of life journey on their mental states. Inspiring a shift in viewpoint creating an atmosphere of change and development.

In the book's concluding moment it resonates an uplifting and inspirational message. Leaving readers inspired to renew passions for their goals towards their mental well-being, empowered by the enlightened knowledge acquired. The conclusion empowers and motivates individuals to become agents of change embarking on their own journeys infused by a deep sense of empathy and courage, radiating with courage and hope.

ENCOURAGEMENT AND HOPE

A Journey Through Mental Health is introduced with a spirit of encouragement and hope. As the narrative reaches the climax readers are embraced in a wave of positivity reaffirming that perseverance is more sore than just an idea, it's a journey. Bringing attention to the essential inner strength within individuals facing mental health challenges, the conclusion unites a broad range of story lines for encouragement. It offers reassurance that every step taken towards understanding and embracing one's mental well-being is a demonstration of courage. Through the stories and interpretation shared, readers discover comfort and regain confidence in their capacity to guide their minds. Hope becomes a guiding light, revealing the direction ahead. The conclusion encourages readers to visualise a future where mental health is approached with kindness, understanding, and acceptance. It prompts a feeling of possibility, reminding individuals that change is not only achievable but a shared responsibility.

In these final pages, the narrative becomes a source of inspiration, motivating readers to embrace hope as a guiding light during challenging times.

The conclusion promotes a sense of assurance that, despite the shadows that may persist, there is always the potential for growth, healing, and a brighter tomorrow. It leaves readers with an intense impression of encouragement and hope, inviting them to carry these opinions forward as they continue their own unique journeys through mental health.

CALL TO ACTION

Readers are urged to apply gained wisdom to effect personal and real world changes. The conclusion empowers individuals to break the silence on mental health through an open conversation and resource promotion This invites readers to embrace the responsibility of support, assisting those on their mental health journeys. It prompts us to confront societal norms, sparking a shared commitment of eradicating shame and encouraging understanding. With a demand for support and guideline improvement, the conclusion inspires readers to become the originator of a mental health environment that supports and accepts every individual.

Empowerment is the guiding principle in the call to action, prompting readers to prioritize self-care, seek professional help when needed, and actively engage in breaking down isolation efforts. As the book comes to an end, it motivates individuals to take action beyond reflection, encouraging them to be an active participant of change in the global conversation surrounding mental health.

The call to action serves as an energetic mentor, transforming the knowledge gained from the journey into meaningful, impactful steps towards a more compassionate and kind hearted globe.

www.ingramcontent.com/pod-product-compliance
Lightning Source LLC
Chambersburg PA
CBHW070948220526
45471CB00007B/2943